Introduction

'Without foundations there can be no fashion', announced the Paris couturier Christian Dior of his much publicised post-war collections in the 1950s. This was certainly true from the eighteenth century to the 1940s, but since Dior wrote those words there has been something of a revolution in the underwear department. It seems that we have thrown modesty to the winds and that underwear has become outerwear. Fashionable clothing has become lighter, briefer and more sheer, and designed to emphasise figures shaped by health and fitness rather than by stays and girdles. Interestingly, underwear styles of the past have influenced designs for contemporary outerwear – Vivienne Westwood's much imitated boned evening bodice and Jean Paul Gaultier's girdle dress are well-known examples.

For women especially the choice is enormous, and worlds away from the end of the nineteenth century when underwear first began to receive attention for its own sake. Underwear provided a comfortable hygienic layer next to the skin, which could be cool and absorbent or keep the wearer warm. It supported and moulded the figure to create the currently fashionable proportion. These foundations also helped to support the shape and weight of the outer garments, and chemises, corset covers and petticoats therefore protected the body from the dress and the dress from the body.

Looking at these sturdy, voluminous objects today it is hard to imagine that they might ever have been considered sexy; but underwear has another, more complicated function – to enhance the physical desirability of the wearer. The erotic status of a garment is not easy to pin down and cannot be dealt with in depth in a book of this size; contemporary writers and illustrators reveal that what was considered respectable, immodest or erotic has varied widely. Social trends dictated what was worn at particular times of day, whether it was to be seen in public or in private and in what company, as well as the sex and age of the wearer. At different points it has been acceptable to show parts or all of an undergarment, and these glimpses are often decorative, designed to appeal to the aesthetic sense, or to titillate.

The work of many authors has been invaluable in the writing of this book and I would like to acknowledge the recent publications of Alison Carter, Aileen Ribeiro, Lynn Sorge and Janet Kent. I would especially like to thank my colleagues at the National Trust and those who have helped with this project, in particular Alison Carter, Margaret Trump, and Kate Strasdin; special thanks are due to Helen Fewster. Brief though it is, I hope that, like a glimpse of stocking or a flash of petticoat, this book will tantalise the reader enough to explore further.

The Chemise

The simply styled long-sleeved chemise worn by Mrs John Bankes (d.1730) of Kingston Lacy in Dorset is very similar to this rare eighteenth-century linen shift from the Royal Albert Memorial Museum, Exeter (below). The sleeves are drawn into a puff over the shoulder and the wide neckline is gathered by a drawstring of linen tape. Basic undergarments like these could be made at home: in 1798 Jane Austen purchased enough linen to make six shifts at 3s 6d a yard.

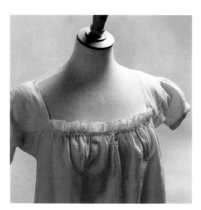

Some of the earliest surviving examples of undergarments are among the most fundamental – the man's shirt, and the woman's smock, shift or chemise. These very basic garments were simply shaped with long sleeves, and sometimes a collar and cuffs, or a drawstring at the neckline to shape and gather the chemise. Sleeves, cuffs and collars prevented heavier outer garments from rubbing and chafing the skin. There seems to have been little differentiation between undershirts and shifts for day and night wear, but class distinctions might be made in the quality of materials used and the type and extent of any decoration.

Linen was preferred for its coolness to touch and its natural absorbency. It also provided a comfortable protective layer between the skin and potentially chafing foundation and over garments. During the sixteenth and seventeenth centuries the wealthy wore the finest linen. *Holland* – the generic name for fine quality fabric that originally came from Holland – was considered the best; when trimmed it might be embroidered or edged with lace, and sometimes both were used to extraordinarily rich effect.

The collar and cuffs of the man's shirt were most likely to be decorated as they were on outward display, less was seen of a woman's chemise, but portraits of the seventeenth and early eighteenth centuries show how the often plain but voluminous chemise sleeves and neck frill were revealed beneath outer garments. By the eighteenth century, men's shirt frills could be extravagantly trimmed with lace, while only the upper frill and sometimes the sleeves of a woman's chemise were visible. As the century progressed the sleeves of the woman's chemise became shorter, and no longer visible beneath the outer garment. Instead engageantes, ruffles of worked muslin or lace, were added at the wrist. Fine, white linen and lace had to look immaculate and was the hallmark of the lady or gentleman.

By the middle of the eighteenth century, the making of underlinen had developed into a specialist trade. In *L'Art de la Lingère* (1771) F.A. de Garsault describes the manufacture and sale of linen in France. The lingère supplied the fabric and specialised in making up undergarments such as shifts and shirts. In England, it was the milliner who provided linen and lace as well as other accessories, such as hosiery and ribbons. As *The London Tradesman* noted in 1747, 'the Milliner furnishes them with Holland, Cambrick, Lawn and Lace of all sorts and makes these Materials into Smocks, Aprons, Tippits, Handkerchiefs, Neckaties, Ruffles, Mobs, Caps, Dressed-Heads with as many Etceteras as would reach from Charing-Cross to the Royal Exchange'.

✓
o6

Inside Out

A Brief History of Underwear

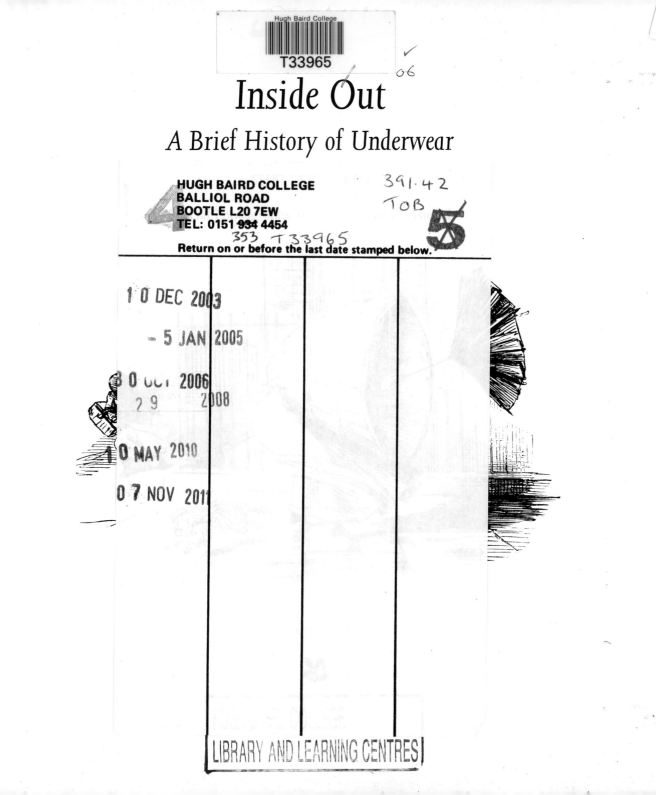

IN MEMORY OF FRANCES TATTERSFIELD (1959–1997)

First published in Great Britain in 2000 by
the National Trust (Enterprises) Ltd
36 Queen Anne's Gate, London SW1H 9AS
www.nationaltrust.org.uk/bookshop

ISBN 0 7078 0370 5

A catalogue record for this book is available from the British Library

Edited by Helen Fewster
Designed and typeset by Peter and Alison Guy
Production by Peter Thompson and Dee Maple
Colour Origination by Colourwise Ltd
Printed in Italy by G. Canale & C.S.p.A

Front cover: The C.B. Corset c.1890 made by Charles Bayer & Co of London Wall on an original shop display stand.
Title page: A Sketch During the Recent Gale appeared in Punch on 20 December 1856, providing
a revealing insight into the crinoline and its management.
Back cover: The actress Pauline Joran's quilted petticoat c.1900 from the Killerton Costume Collection,
an early example of the use of colour in underwear.

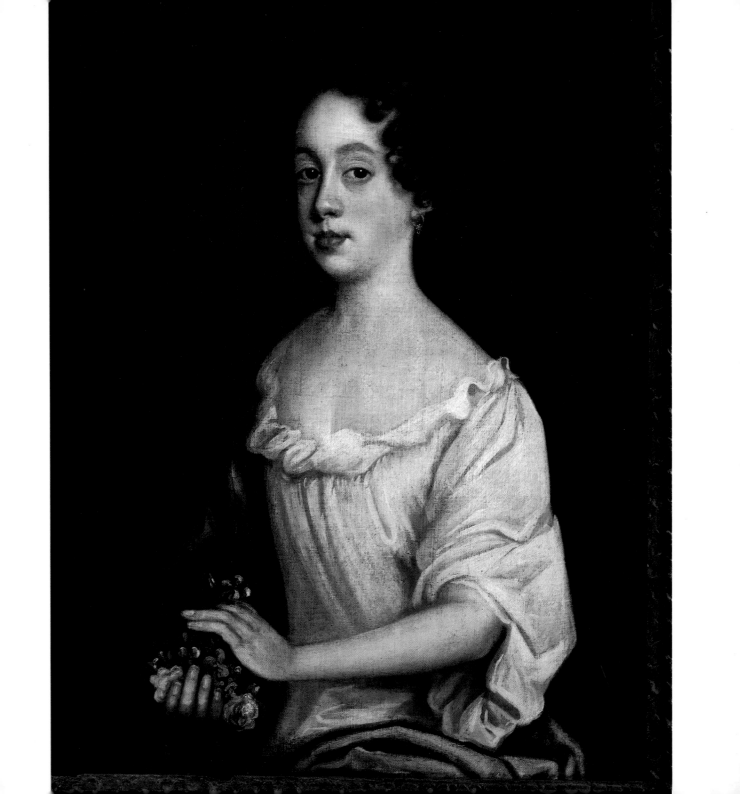

Stays

Lacing up stays similar to the mid-eighteenth-century example shown below was a major operation that required assistance. Despite campaigns from dress reformers, who published articles such as 'An Edict against the use of Stays' in the Lady's Monthly Museum (1800), the fashion for tight lacing continued, providing ample material for caricaturists such as 'Paul Pry', whose New Machine for Winding up the Ladies (right) appeared in c.1828.

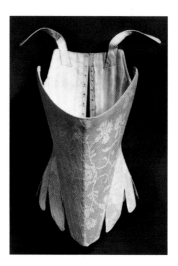

Staymaking was a specialist occupation. During the eighteenth century it was an exclusively male profession because, according to R. Campbell in *The London Tradesman*, 'the Work is too hard for Women, it requires more strength than they are capable of to raise Walls of Defence about a Lady's Shape'. The fitting especially required a delicacy of technique, bearing in mind the potential for immodest revelations or embarrassing situations. As Campbell wrote, the staymaker was therefore required to be:

> a very polite tradesman…and possessed of a tolerable Share of Assurance and Command of Temper to approach their delicate Persons in fitting on their Stays, without being moved or put out of Countenance. He is obliged to inviolable Secrecy in many Instances, where he is obliged by Art to mend a crooked Shape, to bolster up a fallen Hip, or distorted shoulder…to him she reveals all her natural Deformity, which she industriously conceals from the fond Lord, who was caught by her slender Waist.

Stays consisted of several layers of stout canvas or twilled materials woven from linen or cotton threads. This was stiffened with paste and specially shaped sections were stitched together. Different lengths of cord, cane or whalebone, which was favoured for its strength and flexibility, were inserted into hollow casings to help mould the torso and bust, and there was usually a centre front pocket for a wooden busk. Lacing varied and in some cases the garment laced at both back and front to control the shape of the torso and span of the waist. Side lacing was used for stout figures or during pregnancy. Corsets were generally cut low and wide across the bust and were equipped with shoulder straps that also fastened with laces. Soft bindings were added to the bust and armholes – these kid edges were vital for comfort.

Stays might also be worn by army officers, fops and dandies to promote a smart appearance. George IV, as Prince Regent, is famously supposed to have worn them; 'Prinny has left off his stays and his belly now hangs over his knees' wrote Creevey cruelly. Young children of the upper classes were literally moulded by wearing stays to improve their carriage. For the young there was less boning, and possibly less stiffening. Nevertheless, as Elizabeth Ham recalled, her first half-boned stays of c.1792–3, made agonising wearing: 'the first day of wearing them was very nearly purgatory, and I question if I was sufficiently aware of the advantage of a fine shape to reconcile me to the punishment'.

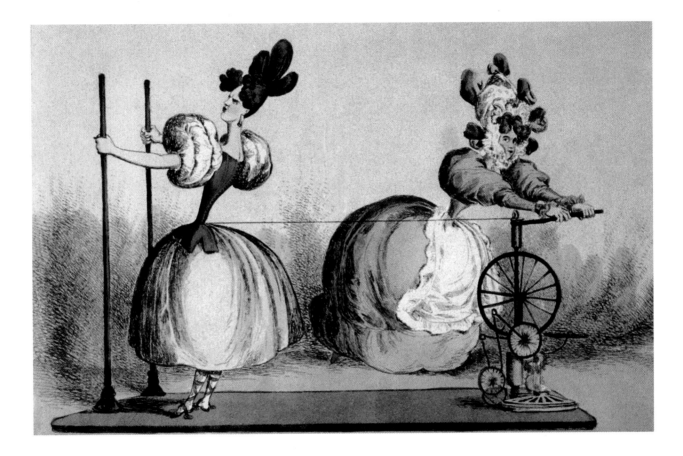

Side Hoops and Bustles

In the early eighteenth century, side hoops or *paniers* were worn over the chemise to support the dress. Hoops were first recorded in 1709 and took the form of satin, linen or cotton petticoats with cane or whalebone inserts. The fashion allowed ladies to wear elaborate gowns at Court which displayed great expanses of luxurious silks in their voluminous skirts. By the 1740s, side hoops were so wide that flexible hoops supported by whalebone were introduced to allow ladies to pass through doorways. Drawstrings helped the wearer to adjust her petticoat, but the oblong shape was difficult to manage, as the *London Magazine* noted in 1768: 'I have been in a moderate large Room where there have been but two Ladies, who had not Space enough to move without lifting up their Petticoats higher than their Grandmothers would have thought decent'.

Despite the tantalising glimpse of ankle afforded as the skirts swung, there was much masculine opposition to this extreme fashion. In 1711, the *Spectator* reported, 'I find several Speculative Persons are of Opinion that our Sex has of late Years been very Saucy, and that the Hoop Petticoat is made use of to keep us at a Distance.' A letter to the *Guardian* in 1713 described the many 'inconveniences' caused by it, such as 'hurting men's shins'. Other inelegant disasters were repeated 140 years later when the crinoline was in vogue: 'I saw a young lady fall down the other day, and believe me, Sir, she very much resembled an over-turned bell without a clapper.'

By the mid-eighteenth century the extreme width of the skirt was retained for full dress only. Instead side hoops were worn tied around the waist with a tape for 'undress' until the mid-1770s. As fashion came to favour gowns with back drapery, hoops were superseded by rumps, a form of bustle. Hip pads were also worn; like rumps they could be made of cotton, wool, padded fabric, or even of cork, which was presumably comparatively light to wear. The Duchess of Devonshire reputedly wore a cork rump back to front to disguise a pregnancy, and set a Court fashion.

The effect could be striking, as Horace Walpole wrote in a letter of 1783:

She was without any stays and being quite free from such an encumbrance the fine play of her easy shape was exhibited in a very advantageous light. She had nothing on but a white muslin chemise, tied carelessly with celestial blue bows; white silk slippers and slight silk stockings…Her hair hung in ringlets down to the bottom of her back, and rested upon the unnatural protuberance which every fashionable female at present chuses to affix to that part of her person.

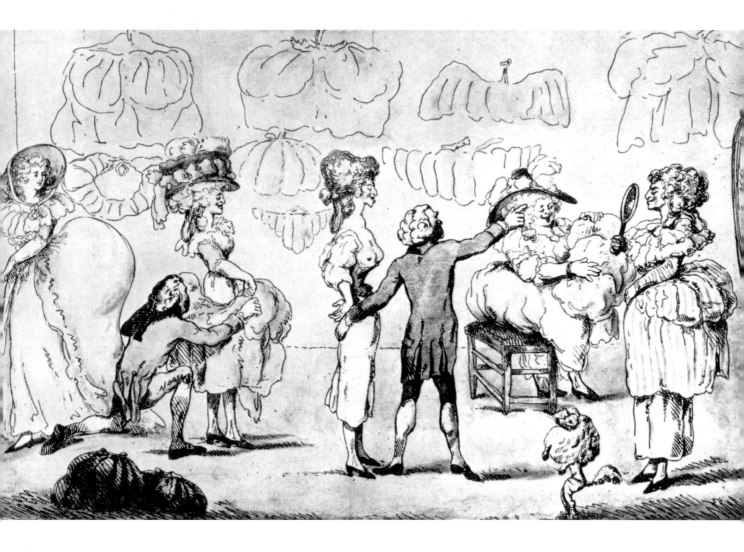

Petticoats

Eighteenth-century images show that a simple knee- or calf-length linen or cotton under-petticoat was worn with stays, pockets and a hoop, or hip pads, over the chemise. Quilted petticoats were added for warmth, and during the first half of the century provided additional support for the dress, replacing or supplementing the hoop. 'There is not one of us but has reduced our outward Petticoat to its ancient Sizeable Circumference, tho' indeed we retain still a Quilted one underneath, which makes us not altogether uncomfortable to the Fashion' reported the *Spectator* in 1711.

These quilted silk or satin petticoats were purely functional and not intended to be seen. Petticoats remained concealed until the open robe revealed decoratively stitched underskirts with elaborate embroidery. Although bulky stiffened petticoats replaced the need for hoops, they could be just as awkward to wear; in 1739 Mr Purefoy returned a quilted petticoat to Long's warehouse because it was too heavy for his sixty-seven-year-old mother. 'You must send a neat white quilted Callico petticoat for my Mother, which must be a yard and four inches long…The Marseilles Quilt petticoat is so heavy my Mother cannot wear it', he wrote.

By the late eighteenth century the increased popularity of the round robe and chemise dress of light transparent muslin had created the need for similarly light undergarments. Full-length petticoats were now worn, sometimes specially made to complement the cut and construction of the dress. Cotton and linen were still used, with flannel providing winter warmth. Dress historians have claimed that the extreme styles of the French 'merveilleuses', who also left off their stays, had little need for underwear, and dampened the muslin drapery so that it clung to the figure. 'Some of our fair dames appear, in summer and winter, with no other shelter from sun or frost than one single garment of muslin or silk over their chemise – if they wear one! … The indelicacy of this mode need not be pointed out; and yet, O shame! It is most generally followed'.

One cannot quite imagine such a fashion having a great following in Britain's chillier and more conservative climate, but stockinette petticoats and a kind of tubular combination garment were apparently available to provide the look of nudity more decently. 'The only sign of modesty in the present dress of the Ladies is the pink dye in their stockings, which makes their legs appear to blush for the total absence of petticoats' reported the *Chester Chronicle* disapprovingly in 1803. Nevertheless, muslins and diaphanous gauzes remained popular, and must have left very little room beneath them for heavy corsetry and petticoats.

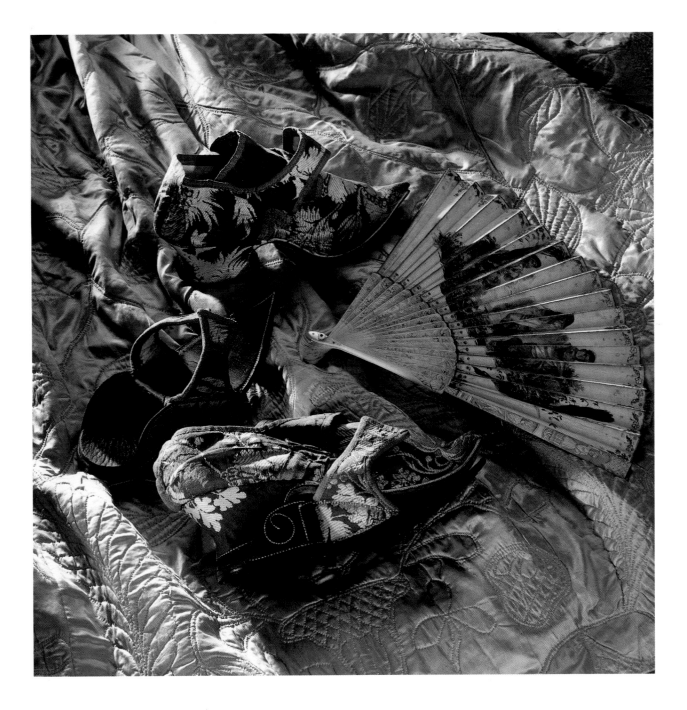

Drawers

Pantaloons and drawers for women seem to have been introduced from c.1800 in response to the sheer dress materials and the 'naked' fashions; there are contemporary references to flesh coloured pantaloons seen under sheer garments worn by an actress on stage. Lady Glenbevie's journal records that the 'modern' and 'sporty' Princess Charlotte was wearing drawers in c.1811. When Lady de Clifford observed that the Princess 'shewed her drawers' and that they were 'much too long', the Princess argued that the Duchess of Bedford's were longer, and 'bordered with Brussels lace'. '"Oh," said Lady de Clifford… "if she is to wear them, she does right to make them handsome."'

However, drawers were not generally adopted by women for some time. In 1841 *The Handbook of the Toilet* recommended them as a French fashion of '…incalculable advantage to women preventing many of the disorders and indispositions to which British females are subject. The drawers may be made of flannel, calico or cotton, and should reach as far down the leg as possible without their being seen'.

Initially pantaloons may have been a childhood fashion, perhaps derived from male clothing. Young boys had been wearing trousers with a short jacket, or a 'skeleton suit' – top and trousers buttoned together – in the 1770s. Separate trouser linings might be made since 'underwaistcoats and drawers were not then worn…' according to Mrs Papendiek, writing in 1790 of her four-year-old son's breeching.

Gentlemen, on the other hand, had worn breeches linings and drawers made of linen or a knitted woollen fabric like stockinette for hygiene, protection and warmth throughout the eighteenth century. An inventory of 1780 reveals that Samuel Curwen, a Massachusetts merchant living in England, possessed 'four pairs of linen drawers, three pairs of leather drawers and one pair of flannel'.

Basic undergarments like drawers and chemises remained loose and simply shaped, and were often made at home, usually from linen or cotton. At first drawers were made of two tubular pieces of fabric to cover the legs, attached to a deep waistband. They were laced at the back and tied with tapes, sometimes brought round to fasten with a button at the front waist for security. Later they became more decorated, usually of plain cambric or longcloth with very reserved whitework embroidery, and pin tucks at hems. Later examples often fasten at the back with a button or tape, and back flap openings and closed legs appeared in the 1870s.

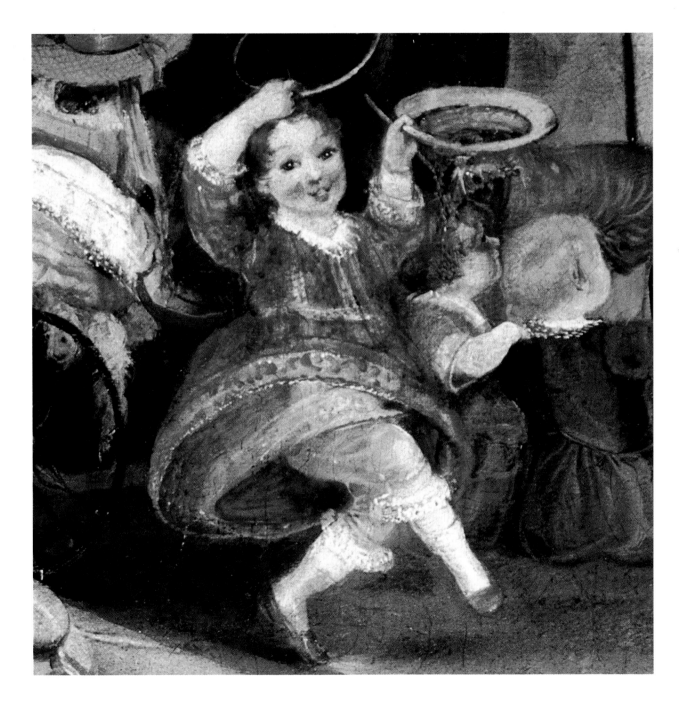

Crinolines and Hoops

An artificial crinoline made by W.S. Thompson and Co. of Cheapside, London, c.1860, shown with a red coutil corset over a chemise. Thompson was a leading manufacturer — their factory produced up to 4,000 crinolines a day — and registered many of their designs, such as the 'Crown' (1866–8) and the 'Winged Jupon' (1868). This example is labelled 'Thompson's, Favourite of the Empress', possibly a reference to Empress Eugènie of France.

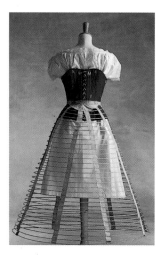

It is hard to believe that the introduction of the hooped petticoat, patented in 1856, was regarded as a boon to women, but it replaced the need for layers of stiffened, corded and woven thread and horsehair petticoats — the original crinoline. Skirts had increased in width from the 1830s, and in *rondeur* throughout the 1840s, so that by the next decade the wearer was surrounded by a multitude of petticoats, with as many as sixteen being worn for Court evening dress. Technological innovations, such as the development of rubber and of fine steels for watch springs, which could be produced on a large scale, provided new materials for superior garments. Some support designs such as the inflatable rubber 'hoop' were registered or patented to prevent piracy.

But perhaps more than any other fashion, the crinoline attracted ribald and outraged comments in equal number. Some of the more racy cartoons and images of the period reveal the instability and undulation of the hoop and all above it was the cause of embarrassing and dangerous incidents. *Punch* and other periodicals published damning articles and caricatures; indeed, Queen Victoria pronounced hoops to be 'indelicate, extravagant' and reputedly refused to wear them until 1868, when she was forced to replace layers of petticoats with a hoop because of the extraordinary heat of that summer.

Swaying and lilting skirts were also a fire hazard as Lady Dorothy Nevill found to her cost:

> I was showing a lady an engraving of Mr Cobden, which he had just given me, and which hung near the fireplace. Somehow or other my voluminous skirt caught fire, and in an instant I was ablaze, but I kept my presence of mind, and rolling myself in the hearthrug, by some means or other eventually beat out and subdued the flames.... None of the ladies present could of course do much to assist me, for their enormous crinolines rendered them almost completely impotent to deal with the fire, and had they come very close to me, all of them would have been ablaze too.

In spite of this, the fashion for the crinoline lasted for nearly twenty years. It spread to all levels of society, and was so hazardous that in 1860 the textile manufacturing firm Courtaulds were forced to announce: 'The present ugly fashion of Hoops or Crinolines as it is called is, however, quite unfitted for the work of our Factories.... We now request our hands at all Factories to leave Hoop and Crinoline at Home'.

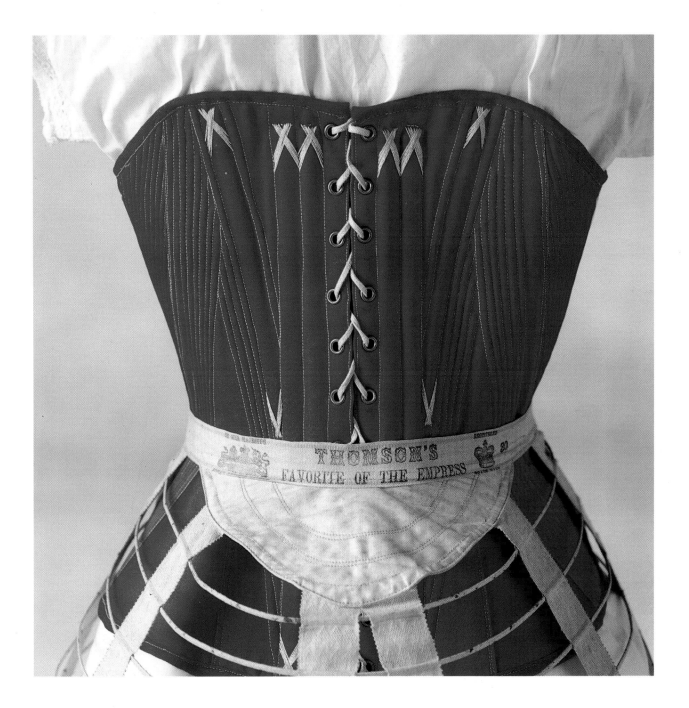

Underwear and Nightwear for Babies and Children

❧

Babies and children's undergarments were usually made of plain white linen or cotton, and woollen fabrics were used for warmth – wool flannel was popular for petticoats and vests. Few of these garments survive because of their practical nature and materials, and attacks from insects. However, as much of the infant wardrobe would have been made at home, many examples are described and illustrated in nineteenth- and early twentieth-century magazines and instruction manuals such as *The Workwoman's Guide* (1838) and weekly publications like the *Englishwoman's Domestic Magazine*.

The preparation of a layette for a newborn baby demanded as much consideration as a trousseau. A properly equipped nineteenth-century baby had a quilted stayband and binders (remnants of swaddling from earlier centuries), nappies, pilches, drawers, pantalettes, combinations, stockings, nightclothes, barras and caps of various materials. Advertisements hint at the huge outlay for the new baby. The Army and Navy Stores catalogue of 1907 recommended a £14 layette of sixty-seven items including nine shirts and eleven swathes or bands of linen and flannel.

As children grew, they would require garments not unlike miniature versions of adult clothes. Stays were worn from an early age, and during the 1860s young girls wore their own shortened version of the cage crinoline, with frilled and embroidered petticoats, long drawers and often brightly coloured patterned stockings showing beneath. According to the *Englishwoman's Domestic Magazine* in 1862, 'A little boy four years old should wear Knickerbockers and petticoats; above that age, Knickerbockers with jackets and waistcoats. Petticoats are worn with a Garibaldi shirt'.

During the twentieth century, firms like Chilprufe of Leicester became leading suppliers of children's clothing, and were particularly known for soft woollen underclothing 'ensuring daintiness, durability, and comfort'. The Chilprufe fabric was claimed to be easily washed and unshrinkable, and because of its silk-like quality the copy went on to state that 'all children who wear Chilprufe are Happy, Healthy, and Contented'. Many people remember differently, recalling scratchy, itchy, uncomfortably hot home-made woollen vests and the restrictions of the Liberty bodice. Symington's Liberty Bodice was born in 1908 as a hygienic and comfortable alternative to stays as it still supported the young figure, but was washable. Made of a fleece-backed cotton jersey fabric, it was reinforced with cotton tapes onto which were sewn 'mangle-proof' rubber buttons to hold petticoats and suspenders in place. It remained a best seller up to the Second World War when shortages restricted its availability.

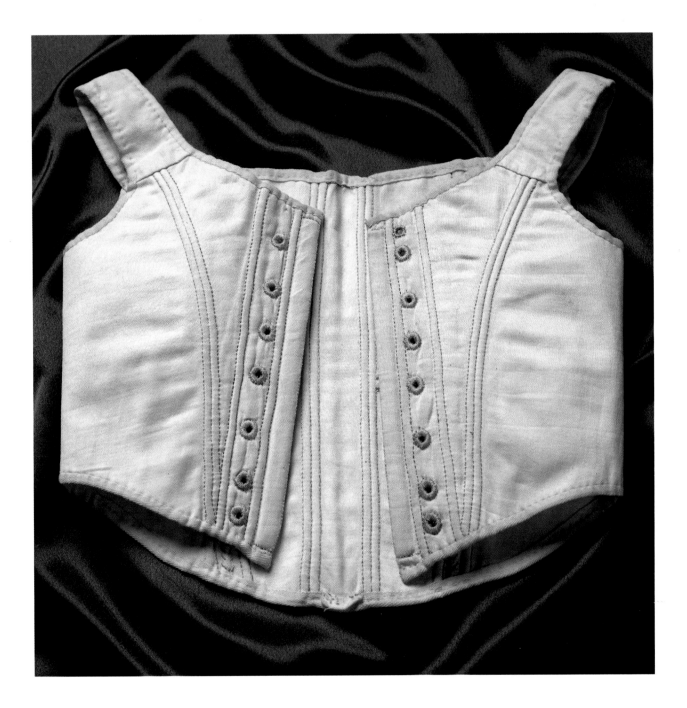

Corsets

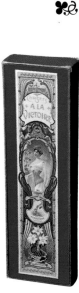

Oh, the pleasure of tight-lacing,
I that have tried, can tell;
Besides that, as to the figure,
I feel I'm quite a belle.
This is the teaching of my lay,
Lace tightly while you can;
Be sure you'll soon forget the pain
You feel when you began.

– Anon, *Englishwoman's Domestic Magazine*, 1869

By the mid-nineteenth century ready-made corsets were widely available, and various claims were made as to their efficacy and 'hygiene'. In the 1830s Mrs Bell, 'Corset maker to Her Highness the Duchess of Kent', produced a 'Regenerating and Sleeping Ceinture' for maternity and post-natal use which 'prevents flatulency, reduces protuberance, supports the stomach and bowels, relieves dropsical symptoms'.

Corsets were available for every figure and occasion, and for most activities, such as riding, considered appropriate for women. Experiments were made with front fastening stays, which were quicker to put on and take off, and by the 1850s the split busk was invented. Made of metal, one side had a series of studs that locked into specially shaped corresponding eyelet holes.

During the 1840s and 1850s stays were laced tighter than ever, and the practice sparked off concern for women's health. In response, staymakers attempted to devise 'healthier' garments. Maternity corsets generally had front lacing from hem to waist which could be let out as the baby grew, and it was recommended that the busk should be removed. During the 1880s the 'Spoon' busk was developed which supposedly put less pressure on the abdomen.

More flexible alternatives to whalebone, such as quillbone and coraline, were also promoted and by the 1900s, metal was replacing natural materials for boning stays. Vollers of Portsmouth introduced the 'Hercules' unbreakable spiral steels, and Spirella continued to use a similar type of steel bone into the 1960s. Steam moulding also helped to give corsets their shape from the 1880s. The garment was applied with a wet starch and heated on a specially shaped block. Charles Bayer of London Wall claimed in *The Ladies' Field* in 1905 that his corsets '…are as easy fitting as a perfectly-cut kid glove…a complete absence of pressure upon the respiratory organs'.

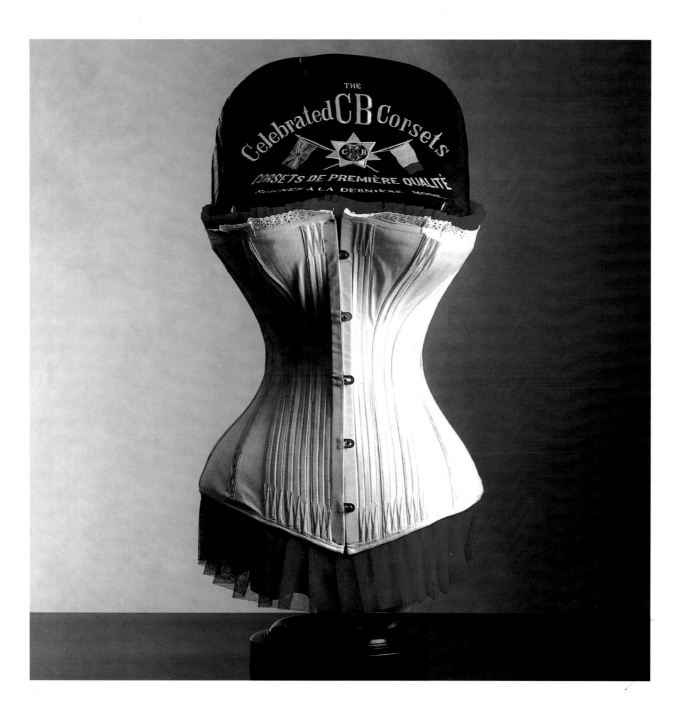

Stockings, Garters and Suspenders

Stockings for men and women, from the seventeenth to the nineteenth centuries showing their decorative clocks. They plainly had an erotic appeal, and the girl on a swing was the subject of many paintings. According to the Spectator in 1712, 'The lover who swings his lady is to tie her clothes very close together with his hat band before she admits him to throw up her heels so that he cannot tell the colour of her garters.' This detail is from Philippe Mercier's painting of the Tyrconnel family of Belton House in Lincolnshire.

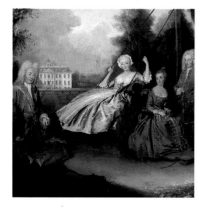

Stockings could be cut from cloth, knitted or woven to shape, and by the beginning of the eighteenth century knitted stockings from wool, cotton or silk threads had replaced cut cloth hose. Some were serviceable and unlovely; others were highly decorative. The finest were of silk, often with beautifully embroidered 'clocks', the decoration at the ankles, drawing attention to the legs. White stockings – mimicking nudity – were particularly fashionable in the 1730s. Lord Kildare of Carton bought elaborately clocked stockings for his wife, Emily, on his trips to London: 'I find I exceed your commission in regard to your stockings with coloured clocks. I bespoke two pairs with bright blue, two pairs with green and two pairs with pink clocks…. I am sure when you have them on your dear legs will set them off…the writing about your stockings and your dear, pretty legs makes me feel what is not to be expressed'.

At first stockings were gartered just above or below the knee with a decorative ribbon. The ribbons themselves are of interest for they might be woven with slogans, such as 'God Save the King' marking the return of George III after his illness in the 1780s. By the 1800s decorative suspenders – independent garters – were worn, like the chenille embroidered spring garter. Suspender belts were introduced in 1887 – the London firm L. Hoven and Co. advertised the 'Improved Patent Stocking Suspender', similar to modern versions, as entirely superseding garters, and suitable for all sexes and ages. Sock suspenders were available for men. Suspenders were also added to corsets towards the end of the nineteenth century; innovations included Kleinert's hook-on hose supporters (1902) which clipped to the front edge of the corset.

Chemical dyes were developed from the 1850s, and by the early twentieth century stockings were available in a myriad of colours, even purple, green and canary yellow, like the 'thick silk stockings, vermilion, cornflower blue and grey, bought in Paris' that D.H. Lawrence described in *Women in Love*. Harrods' catalogue of 1900 includes stockings of 'black cotton with white feet' to prevent feet staining black in hot weather.

In 1902, only coloured embroidery was deemed acceptable by the sophisticated, and some women matched their stockings to their shoes. Mrs Eric Pritchard referred to bronze or black with self-coloured clocks as being the most fashionable in this year – 'a "gay" stocking may be excusable in some instances, but it is not to be catalogued in the really fashionable hosiery of the hour'. Taupe, gunmetal, brown and black were the colours most often worn, but by the early 1920s flesh and skin tones had also been introduced. They were made in lisle, silk and artificial silk, or rayon, a fabric developed by the firm Du Pont.

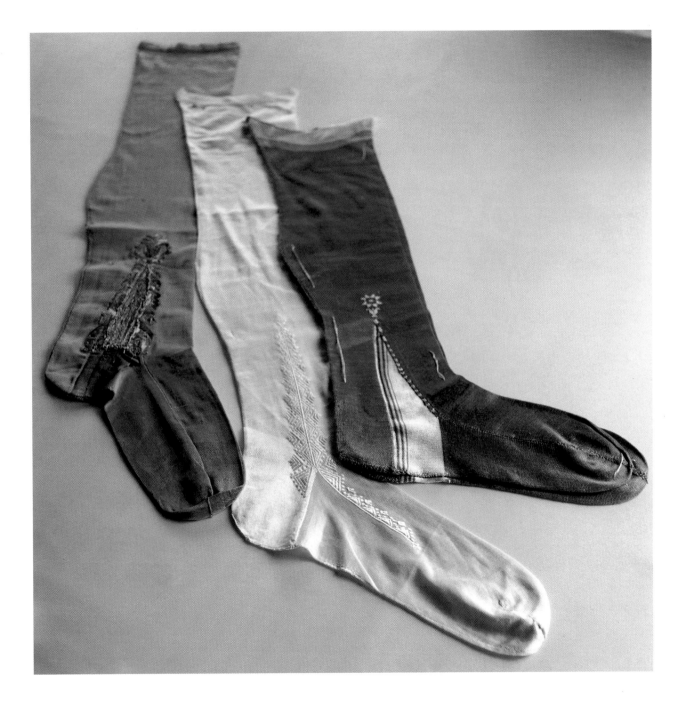

Crinolettes and Bustles

By the 1870s fashions had changed: the crinoline was superseded by a new shape created by tournures – bustles – and the crinolette. This was made from half hoops of whalebone inserted into plain or striped muslin and suspended from a waistband tied with tapes. More complicated versions incorporate lacing to help control the shaping mechanism. Smaller tournures were made from a variety of materials, including wool and horsehair, and frames of metal. In 1879 *The Queen* described the new look:

> They are made of steel and thick muslin; some reach almost to the hem of the dress…a great deal depends on the figure; but many Frenchwomen wear only a small dress improver just on the bend of the back, more a pad than anything else, to which is attached three short flounces of washing silk, corded throughout, by which I mean thick cords are run in to give the silk substance; and each flounce is box pleated. They require frequent renewing….The dress improvers are much worn by those who are particular about the set of their skirts, and are made to order; but the striped muslin made to tack into the back of the skirt, is also used…. Black muslin is used for dark dresses, white for the light.

'Why revive the old wire fencing, though you call it crinolette?' grumbled *Punch* in 'The Chant of the Crinolette' in 1881. Despite such opposition, the new tournure was regarded as a stylish necessity, as *Myra's Journal* reported in the same year. 'Letters pour in with queries as to the necessity for wearing the tournure, and all kinds of hopes and fears are expressed as to the coming in of crinoline – All fashionable women wear a slight tournure, and even those who hesitate on the brink of a mode, must own the improvement to most figures'.

The selection of an appropriate tournure was a matter of good taste, 'for it must not only suit the dress but the person wearing it'. Instead of just one foundation for all types of skirt, various tournures were worn depending on the type of garment: a long jupon-tournure for evening dress; a small 'puff' for a morning gown; a short tournure for walking. By the mid-1880s, however, they were no longer regarded as so elegant. Their decline was noted in *Myra's Journal* in 1884 with the comment that 'the tournure has reached ridiculous proportions…a too voluminous pouf will destroy the charm of the most elegant toilette.' And by 1888 the magazine was reporting that 'well-dressed women wear scarcely any tournure'.

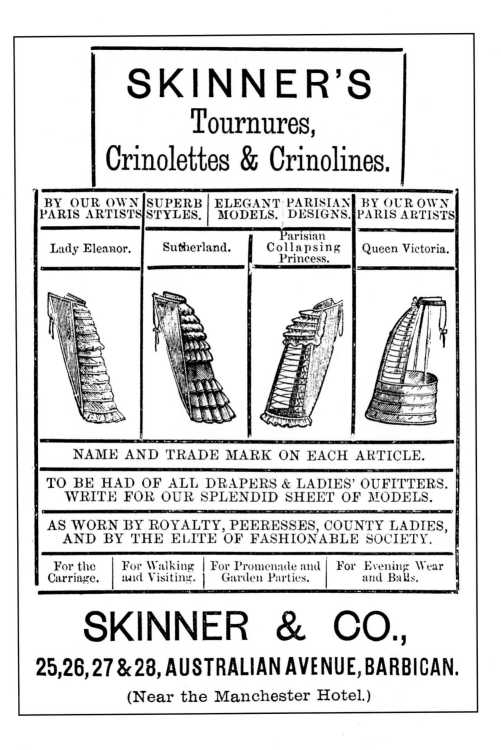

Warmth and Practicality

Quilted petticoats remained popular in the nineteenth century for winter wear, although, unlike the decorative petticoats of a century before, they were not intended to be seen. However, some quite colourful winter undergarments were produced during the 1870s and 1880s; the designs were often registered in an attempt to protect the copyright for there was fierce competition from rival manufacturers. Booth and Fox of London supplied all manner of quilted textiles including bed quilts and their registered down clothing. A newspaper advertisement of c.1877 stresses the healthy benefits of using their 'Patent Real Down Quilts and Skirts'. Underskirts, dressing gowns and vests – a kind of buttoned under bodice – were invaluable for invalids and those of a delicate constitution since 'No cold can penetrate a Down Garment'. One testimonial came from participants in an Arctic expedition who found them 'useful for observers and others who had to stand about much in the cold'; according to 'an Eminent Professor of Chemistry…Messrs Booth and Fox's Down Clothing consists solely of pure, soft, scentless down'.

Innovative all-in-one garments appeared in magazines like the *Girl's Own Paper*. Chemilettes and combinations reduced the need for bulky layers of soft garments under the new fashionably tight fitting sheath dresses of the early 1880s. By this time the Dress Reform movement, which had long opposed tightly laced stays and corsets, was gaining strength. An 1883 edition of *The Queen* contained 'Hints on Dress Reform', having recently noticed 'how needlessly uncomfortable our dress is'. The writer advises reducing the number of bulky layers of undergarments and explains how she made herself a combination garment by adapting drawers and chemise and joining them together. Without this, she says, there is no point in leaving off stays since the ugly waistbands still showed through. She declares that 'some people can look tidy with no stays at all, and they generally wear a close fitting jersey instead; but most women must have some kind of support to the bust, not only for appearance sake, but for health and comfort'.

The campaign for rational dress incorporated an interest in the 'woollen movement', which supported the claims of Dr Gustave Jaeger and his Sanitary Woollen Underwear. Oscar Wilde, himself an advocate of artistic dress, lectured on the subject and George Bernard Shaw wore suits of Jaeger's knitted jersey. Jaeger's first shop was opened in Fore Street in the City of London in 1883. His combination undergarments were rather charmless, but many believed in the wisdom of wearing wool next to the skin, not only to keep warm but to absorb perspiration.

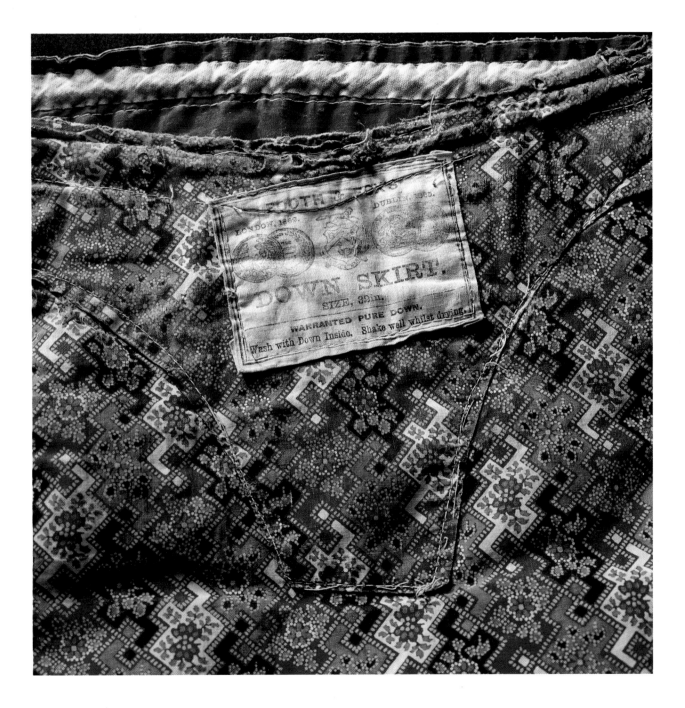

Nightwear and Undress

A man's brown satin dressing-gown, c.1830, embroidered with silks in bird and flower motifs. This was an acceptable form of undress for men, as this detail (below) from an 1857 fashion plate shows: a gentleman receives his guests in a dressing-gown and smoking cap.

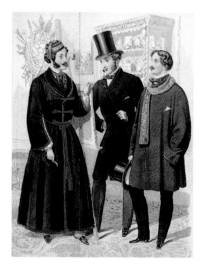

The blurred distinctions between underwear, undress and nightwear can sometimes cause confusion especially when looking at seventeenth- and eighteenth-century dress. In essence, these garments were not seen in public, but the term undress usually distinguishes informal from formal full dress clothes. Some forms of undress would never have been seen outside the home or boudoir, although they were considered decent and fashionable enough to be worn in the company of one's family or closest friends. Indeed, during the eighteenth century many men sat for portraits in banyans (a kind of fitted dressing-gown) worn over a shirt, and indoor caps without formal wigs. These were usually made of rich and expensive fabrics, such as silk damask, and could be extravagantly embroidered. By the middle of the nineteenth century this relaxed dress was replaced by full length dressing-gowns and short smoking jackets and caps. For women, the morning ritual of the toilette demanded a suite of pretty but protective clothing in the form of wrapping gowns and peignoirs (literally for wear when dressing the hair). By the 1920s, these fairly modest garments were replaced by silky negligée and kimono style dressing gowns accessorised with boudoir caps.

As for nightwear, in earlier periods there seems to have been little differentiation between what was worn right next to the skin in or out of bed. By the early nineteenth century there were more definite distinctions between day and night shifts, although they were still of simple construction and worn with cotton or woollen nightcaps to keep out the chill night air which some believed caused disease. There were apparently some who preferred to envelop the body completely – one young bride was so horrified by seeing her husband in his short nightshirts that she decided to spend her honeymoon 'making him nice long night-gowns so that I shan't be able to see any of him'.

By the 1890s, pyjamas were replacing the nightshirt, although the latter was still produced and worn well into the twentieth century. Striped flannels and silks were particularly popular for men's pyjamas, but they were also available for women in a more decorative version with lace or embroidery trimmed collars. Janet Walker of Regent Street advertised ladies' pyjamas in pure wool 'in a variety of dainty colours' in *Madame* in 1901. The accompanying illustration shows a beribboned and flounced tunic with long sash over harem style trousers gathered at the ankles. However, pyjamas did not become universally popular for women until the 1920s and full length, long-sleeved, high-necked nightgowns prevailed. Many examples – often of the stout cotton cambric variety – survive in museum collections.

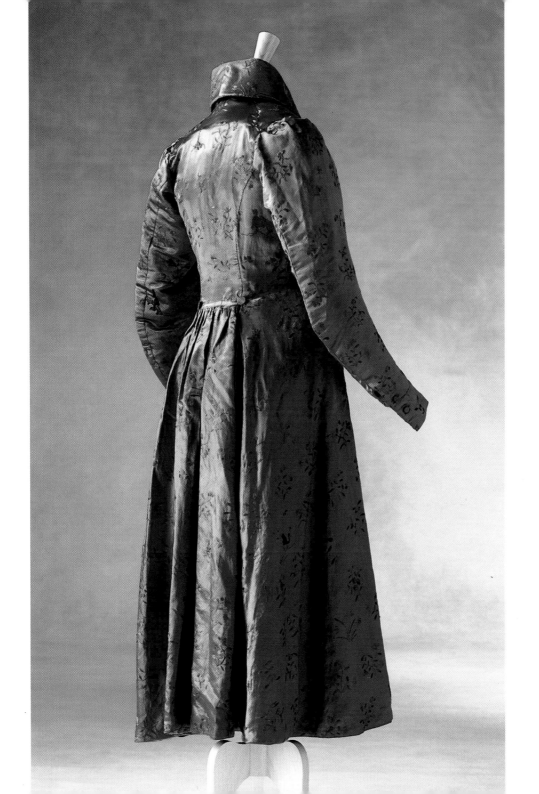

The Trousseau

The trousseau was perhaps one of the major areas of discussion in feminine dress in the nineteenth century, and underwear comprised an important part of it. Most women reserved their prettiest and most decorative underwear for it. It could involve a relatively large outlay, as the advice offered by the *English Woman's Domestic Magazine* to a bride endeavouring to practise economy in May 1862 reveals: 'Marion. By reducing the number of articles in the Trousseau, and having six instead of 12 of different things, you will arrive at something suitable for your income.'

The innovative ladies' and children's outfitter Mrs Bauer offered 'Novel and Perfect Shapes in Hand-made Underclothing for Trousseaux' for which she was awarded two prize medals at the Paris Exhibition of 1878. Her combined system of cutting produced a registered design for a combination garment adapted for hot weather which the *Daily Telegraph* felt 'might win the cordial approbation of a sanitary reformer'.

'In no item of dress has there been more changes in fashion of late years than in underwear. The chief aim now seems to be to minimise all such garments', announced *The Queen* in 1880.

> Washing silk (both cream and coloured) has taken the place of cambric and linen for day and night chemises. White flannel petticoats are things of the past; coloured flannel, with much fancy stitching and torchon lace, has superseded them; also black satin skirts lined with chamois leather. Black satin stays are fast taking the place of white coutil, and stocking suspenders have dethroned garters…and every ingenious contrivance is resorted to for reducing hips and busts, because slim figures remain the mode.

Correspondents to *The Queen* frequently asked for advice on appropriate dress for the colonies. In July 1880, 'Subaltern's Wife' and 'V.C.' were reassured that underlinen could be well made in India and that Indian gauze, merino vests, and fine flannel petticoats were required. 'As regards underclothing, one dozen nightdresses, two dozen chemises, two dozen drawers, is about the usual quantity, made of the thinnest longcloth, of fine, close texture (Horrocks's 'E.F.' is good) trimmed with pretty network or lace. In choosing stockings, V.C. must remember that the mosquitoes are a certain pest, and that, if too thin in texture, they bite through; save for this, Lisle thread and silk can be worn'.

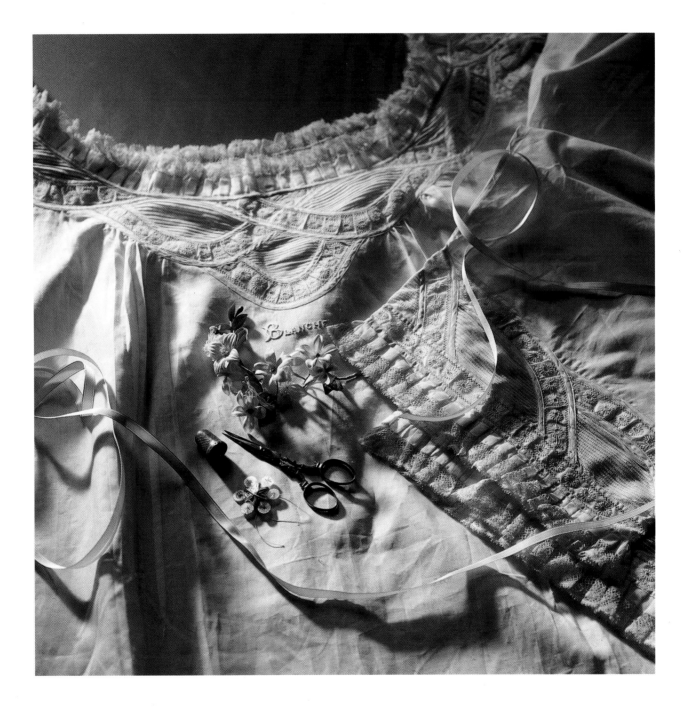

Underwear for Show!

By 1902 the term 'lingerie' no longer seems to refer to the white embroidered accessories to dress such as collars and cuffs, chemisettes and caps, but to beautiful underwear. Writing in *The Cult of Chiffon* (1902), Mrs Eric Pritchard advised that 'exquisite lingerie forms the foundation of the wardrobe of the woman of refinement', suggesting that out of a dress allowance of £200 a year, one-fifth should be put aside for lingerie and corsets.

The introduction and acceptance of coloured fabrics and decoration for underwear began in the late nineteenth century, but its wearing was in general considered rather 'fast'. Coloured silks, embroidered decoration, and lace trimmings adorned stays and corsets and may have invaded the trousseau but did not become more widely worn until the 1900s. For most women underwear was permitted to be practical but not colourful, and certainly never sexy; 'A virtuous woman has a repugnance to excessive luxury in her underclothing', remarked the Baroness Staffa in 1892.

But by the time Mrs Pritchard's book was published, lingerie was definitely intended for display. 'It is in the details of the invisible that refinement is expressed; they give the measure also of woman's sense of beauty; and the woman possessed of the laudable desire to appear lovely in her husband's eyes will not fail, if she be wise in her generation, to give this part of her wardrobe careful consideration'.

The British couturière Lucile was famous for her confections of lace and chiffon, and also supplied delicate lingerie to her clients. In her memoirs, published in the 1930s, she even claimed to have invented the brassière. Her sister, the flamboyant writer Elinor Glyn, refers to similar garments in her novels. In *The Vicissitudes of Evangeline* the innocent heroine's Valenciennes trimmed nightgown of 'fine linen cambric nicely embroidered' and pink silk dressing-gown from Doucet's are a cause for concern amongst her older friends, not because she is in mourning and has not had time to replace the dressing-gown with a more seemly plain white garment, but because the pretty nightgown is not fit 'for a girl – or for any good woman for that matter…(because) no nice-minded woman wants things to look becoming in bed!'

Glyn also sums up the importance of respectable 'frillies' to a fashionable young woman in *The Visits of Elizabeth*: 'The Rooses told me it wasn't 'quite nice' for girls to loll in hammocks (and they sat on chairs) – that you could only do it when you are married; but I believe it is because they don't have pretty enough petticoats. Anyway…as I knew my 'frillies' were all right, I hammocked too, and it was lovely.'

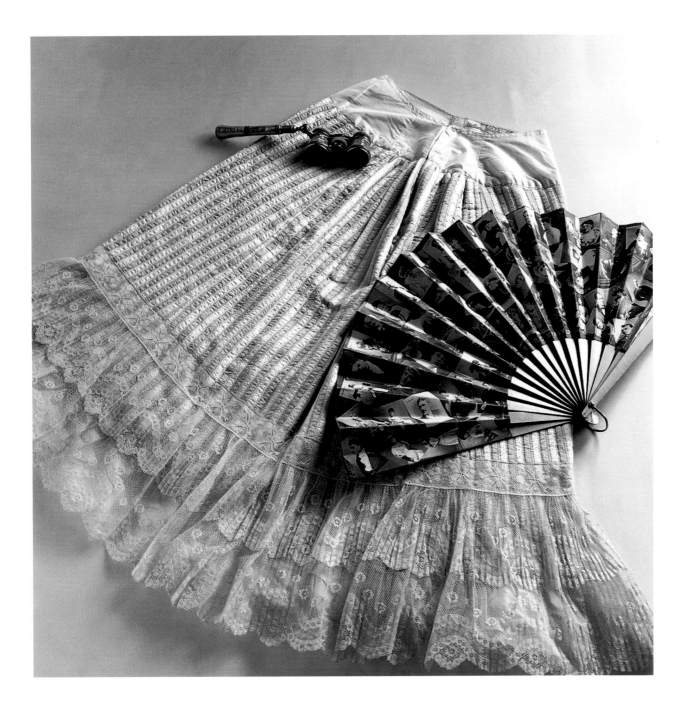

Ready to Wear

Most stores had departments specialising in trousseaux and, indeed, in lingerie for every occasion. 'I was particularly anxious to have a department for beautiful under-clothes, as I hated the thought of my creations being worn over the ugly nun's veiling or linen-cum-Swiss embroidery which was all the really virtuous woman of these days permitted herself', recalled Lucile in her memoirs in the 1930s. 'I started making underclothes as delicate as cobwebs and as beautifully tinted as flowers, and half the women in London flocked to see them, though they had not the courage to wear them at first.'

Stores such as Debenham and Freebody (then at Cavendish House on Wigmore Street and Welbeck Street in London, and the Promenade in Cheltenham) had separate departments for lingerie and hosiery. Mail order catalogues were issued in booklet form and patterns and designs were forwarded free to all parts of the country and to India and the colonies. Their *Fashion Book* of Spring 1870 included designs for 'Novel-ties, Costumes, Mantles, Ball Dresses etc.' with prices and descriptions 'specially intended as an assistance to ladies ordering by post'. Garments were available ready-made as well as from the workrooms. In the case of the best quality underwear 'ready-made' could literally mean hand-stitched as it was not acceptable for 'ladies' to wear anything else.

Other London-based firms such as Bauer of Oxford Street, who specialised in children's clothes and trousseaux, also sent out illustrated catalogues with directions for self-measurement on request. The catalogues included novelty and high fashion garments as well as standard clothing. The 1912 catalogue from Woollands, the Knightsbridge department store, shows a petticoat for tango – 'new petticoat made for the present mode in Ninon with two steels, which are easily removed. The shaped flounce is of Ninon, handsomely embroidered by hand, and inset with Net medallions. Price of model 7 guineas, can be copied with lace flounce from 3 guineas'. Accompanying it in the illustration is a low v-necked camisole of Valenciennes lace, which was suitable for wearing under transparent blouses. An evening camisole of fine net and lace offered at 21/9 has ribbon straps instead of sleeves, presumably so that the undergarment will not show beneath the gown.

Dainty Novelties

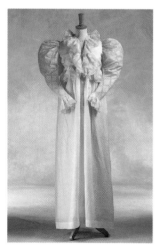

A nightdress of c.1890, which belonged to Pauline Joran. It is extravagantly trimmed with lace, and may have been part of her trousseau.

During the 1900s interest was revived in both antique and modern lace. It featured heavily in the wardrobe, as all kinds of garments were trimmed with different types of hand- and machine-made lace or imitations such as Irish crochet and 'chemical' lace – a form of machine embroidery. Edgings in Torchon and Valenciennes ('Val') patterns were considered particularly appropriate for underclothes; according to a Dickins and Jones catalogue of 1886 'Real Torchon Lace…is the most durable trimming for ladies' and children's underclothing'. Other suitable laces included Point de Paris, 'a New thread Lace, specially adapted for trimming underlinen, very strong and effective' and 'Nursery Embroidery…a most durable article for trimming Children's underwear. Outwears any article it might be attached to'.

There was a huge market for lace, which was stocked by department stores and haberdashers. Often it was produced by charities or convents, and this was emphasised by advertisers: 'Ladies' Underclothing – The Stock, consisting only of high-class Goods made by hand on the premises, by Nuns in Convents, and by Scotch and Irish peasant women, as at all former sales, will be cleared at a great reduction in price. Ladies contemplating matrimony will find this a favourable opportunity for obtaining superior articles at the price of ordinary goods.' In 1902, *Home Chat* revealed that Irish lace was particularly prized:

> Ireland has awoke to find itself famous in the great cause of lace. From every high authority in the land comes the assurance that Irish crochet lace is to carry all before it next season. Great ladies are searching every known record for the designs rendered obsolete by disuse, and the utmost secrecy is observed when some lost treasure is recovered. Many coronation gowns will bear evidence of this latest cult.

A receipt for items from P. Steinmann & Co. of Piccadilly in Exeter's Royal Albert Memorial Museum shows that in 1933 a Miss Colwill paid sixteen shillings for a 'Real Irish Lace chemise Top'. This highlights the distinction made between 'real' and machine or other imitation (e.g. embroidered) laces. The decorative 'top' would be mounted on suitable material either as a dress yoke or perhaps as a camisole.

The often fine and flimsy fabrics used for Edwardian frou-frou and luxury lingerie required special pleating and goffering to keep them looking good. The laundering of undergarments was frequently discussed in women's magazines like *The Queen* and the *Girl's Own Paper*, which carried an article on 'How to get up lace and chiffon' in 1901.

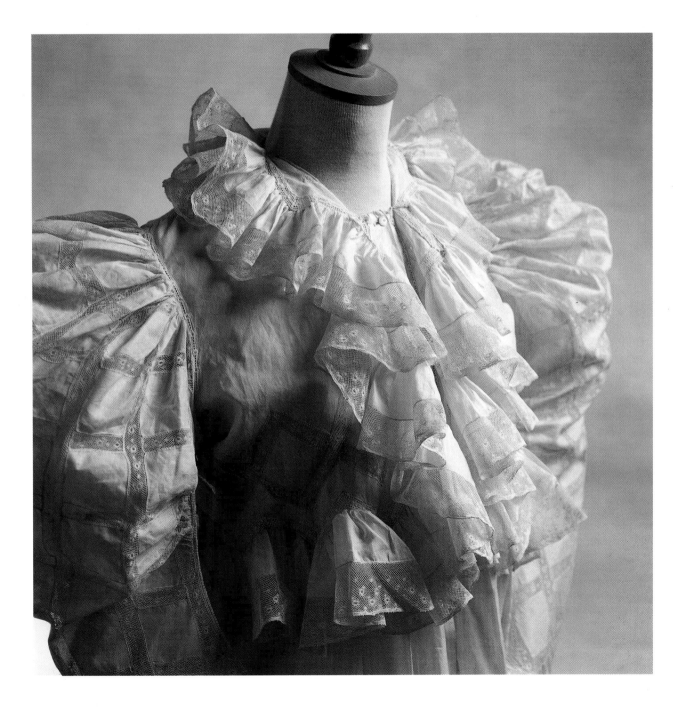

To Corset, or not to Corset...

'Corsets are made straighter fronted than ever. Waists are considered trifles to which all sensible women have said good-bye', announced *The Lady* in October 1902. The corset of the period – the 'S' bend – was tightly laced into the back of the waist, creating a womanly figure with hips thrust back and a 'pouter pigeon' chest.

In general, corsets compressed the bust and hips of women of more generous proportions, but stays were also made to flatter slim figures, such as those sold by the aptly named Madame Lacie of Warwick Street. 'The sides are cut away to encourage hips, and the back, while luxuriously supple, ensures the coveted bend prescribed equally by the canons of Art and Fashion. If desired, a ruching of silk is inserted at the bust to prevent the stay from pressing, and also to help the set of a blouse or bodice. In cases of extreme thinness, this last is a vast improvement, for there is nothing more unfeminine or unattractive than a flat-chested woman.'

The move towards the long slim lines of the high-waisted Directoire style required a different kind of corset. Few were daring enough to follow the couturières' recommendation and leave off their stays altogether; instead they adopted a garment that narrowed the waist and slenderised the hips and upper thighs – a bridge between stays and a girdle. The first bust bodices and bras soon followed. Both the British Lucile, and the American Caresse Crosby, claimed to have 'invented' the brassière, but it is interesting to note that advertisements were already referring to the bust bodice as suitable for wear beneath the more diaphanous garments as early as 1903. 'The Daintily designed, properly-shaped Bust bodices of the London Corset Company give and preserve the beautiful outlines of the perfect figure, indispensable to the wearers of Tea-gowns, Blouses, etc., price 10s. 6d., 19s. 6d.'

The Killerton Collection has several early brassières and bust bodices dating from c.1910 to the 1920s and made from a variety of materials – from stout cotton to flimsy machine lace. The earlier cotton example is embellished simply with broderie anglaise and laces at the back rather like a corset, while the less supportive types are prettily trimmed with ribbons and braid and rosebuds. For 'problem' figures additional help was at hand in the form of a 'bust support', 'one of the most dainty little satin things imaginable' recommended to be worn over the top of the corset to take away 'that "spread" look from a stout figure'. Contemporary mail order catalogues, such as Sears and Roebuck show corset covers with stiffened ruffles to help compensate for nature and increase the dimensions of the bust.

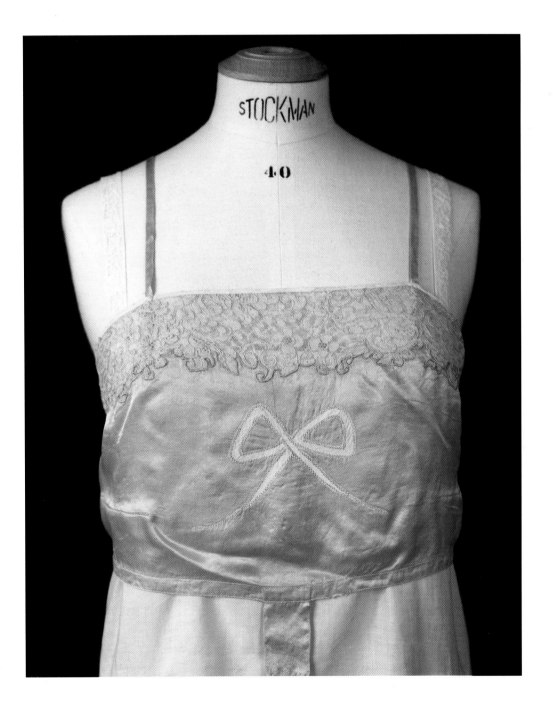

Tea Gowns and Negligées

A Liberty tea gown of c.1897 from Ickworth in Suffolk. It is made of green satin with velvet hanging sleeves, embroidered with flowers in beads and topaz. The inner sleeves and the ruching at the neck are of pale green chiffon.

A form of undress, rather than underclothing or nightwear, the tea gown originated in the 1880s, when artistic and historical versions were produced by the firm Liberty. They were for wear at home, and often made of rich fabrics and based on medieval and renaissance dress. The gowns were usually loose fitting and although they did not require a corset, there must have been many fashionable women who were reluctant to give them up.

The tea gown was intended to allow relaxed dressing in private and came into its own in the 1900s when it was produced in a variety of versions. The sensuous garments created by the couturier Mariano Fortuny, such as his finely pleated silk Delphos dress, were intended to show feminine curves unrestricted by stays. Contemporary photographs of Fortuny's house models record how the soft lines of the ample Edwardian figure were revealed beneath the clinging lines of the dress. Other versions depicted in the pages of fashion and dressmaking magazines were obviously intended for wear over stays lest they appear inelegant. Those that survive are wonderful confections of wispy chiffon and pleated mousseline de soie or jap silk, finely trimmed with lace and delicate embroidery. Short tea-jackets were also produced, and there was a fashion for wearing Oriental gowns and jackets as rest gowns in the boudoir.

In 1902 Mrs Pritchard described the tea gown in *The Cult of Chiffon* as 'a garment of mystery which can be a very complete reflection of the wearer'. The ideal tea gown 'of accordion pleated chiffon, lace and hanging stoles of regal furs' was just one example of the garment which could be worn 'in our own drawing rooms, when the tea-urn sings at five o'clock, we can don these garments of poetical beauty'.

Others found them less attractive. According to Lady Diana Cooper in *The Rainbow Comes and Goes*: 'The ladies dressed for tea in trailing chiffon and lace, and changed again for dinner into something less limp'.

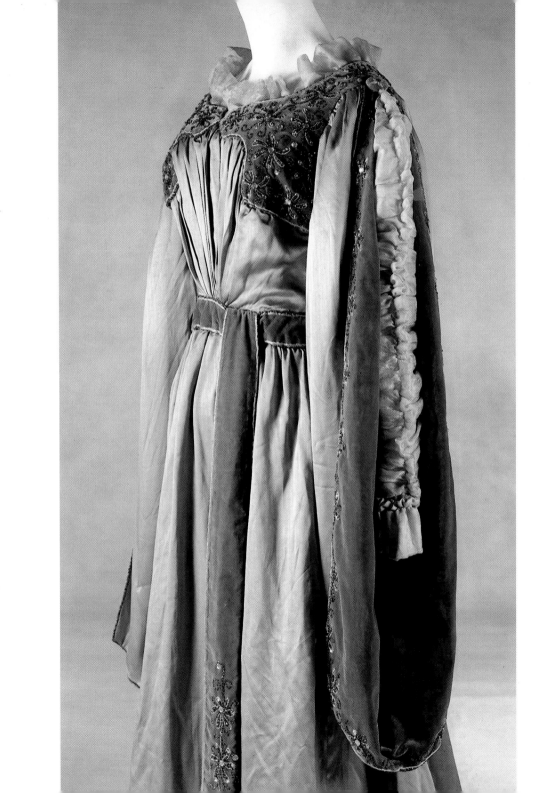

Home-sewn Lingerie

The skills of hand-knitting and plain sewing became increasingly important during the war years. The weekly penny magazine *Our Home* included a regular feature on 'Practical Dressmaking' by 'Ivy'. Free patterns were sometimes provided; the issue of 20 February 1915 included a brown tissue paper pattern for a lady's chemise already cut to shape. Ivy suggested making it up in safe choices of fine longcloth, tarantulle or madopalam – all cottons. It could be decorated with lace, frills or embroidery, but the cut of the chemise was extremely plain, shaped simply at the yoke with rows of pintucks.

Our Home paper patterns were available in small medium and large sizes and were guaranteed to be 'perfectly cut, well shaped and in good style'. The giveaway patterns were featured each week and produced for a medium figure, cut to a 24-inch waist. The sizing systems that we are now accustomed to did not develop until after the Second World War. Women engaged in war work needed to be practical in their dress, while those fighting needed warm and practical undergarments – hence the proliferation of knitting patterns with designs for 'comforts for soldiers'.

Much underwear and nightwear was still home-made in the 1920s and 30s, especially the more traditional cotton variety, and paper patterns were available to help the bride-to-be and new mother make their own trousseaux and layettes. The Women's Institute of Domestic Arts and Sciences invited women to purchase their practical instruction book, which included thirty-eight patterns for lingerie garments. Interest grew in all kinds of craft and needlework that could be easily done at home; crochet was particularly popular. An advertisement for Ardern's crochet threads from *Home Notes* in 1926 underlines the importance of and fascination with the 'bottom drawer': 'Whenever there's a minute to spare she slips softly to her room to admire those fascinating lace things – her own exquisite handiwork'.

Magazines aimed at the mass market and the working girl, such as *Home Notes* and the *Girl's Own Paper*, offered hints on dressmaking and needlework, illustrating practical garments like the envelope chemise whose patterns could be sent for by post. Their readers were unlikely to be able to afford the fashionably luxurious silk and chiffon confections featured in *Vogue* but cheaper coloured fabrics and silk substitutes of varying quality were becoming available. The Manchester firm Tootal's sold patterns for making up its 'guaranteed' textiles through these magazines – for instance 'Tarantulle' was recommended for white and coloured lingerie. Advertisements emphasised that colours would not fade: 'Everything's Tarantulle and you know that's guaranteed.'

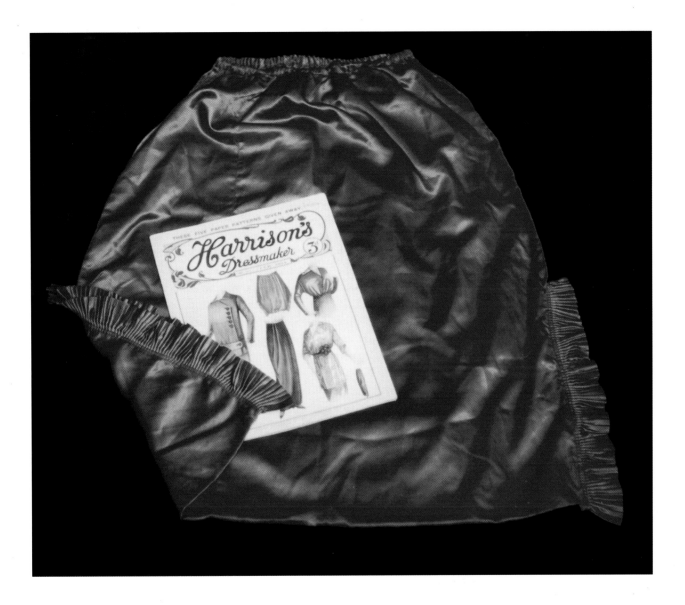

The 1920s

✿

Throughout the 1920s and 1930s girdles and bust flatteners gradually replaced the waist-reducing corsets of previous years. At the same time, new rubber 'reducing' corsets were advertised which were claimed to help the wearer to slim — presumably they were more likely to lose water than fat. Various styles of bra emerged, including Gossard's longline and uplift models. All kinds of materials were used, from traditional batiste to knitted fabrics and rayon, and there was a limited colour range available in suitable 'lingerie' shades, including the ubiquitous white and peach popularised by firms such as Twilfit, Fitu and Spirella.

However, the new synthetics were not always able to compete with Tootal's guaranteed fabrics. They were still rather unstable, and prone to disintegration after much wear and laundering. The Artificial Silk Exhibition of 1926 demonstrated the versatility and appropriateness of rayon for items like women's underwear, but it did not begin to become really popular until the 1930s and 40s, when brands like Mylesta and Ferguson were widely advertised as silk substitutes. The use of fancy or foreign sounding brand names and terms like Art silk enhanced the appeal of what was often an inferior product.

Contemporary magazines and newspapers were now able comfortably to describe and illustrate women's underwear without any of the coyness or modesty of earlier periods. Newspapers like the *Daily Mail* unashamedly carried advertisements for all kinds of goods — even the least glamorous — especially at sale time, as an advert for the London Glove Company promoting 'Startling Offers in Directoire Knickers' shows. 'Nearly 2,000 pairs of GIRLS' really good quality soft close texture stockinette, with fleecy back, DIRECTOIRE KNICKERS, elastic at the waist and knee. These garments will wear well and wash splendidly.'

Equally invaluable in cold weather but just as unglamorous were the elasticated combinations that were now widely available. Killerton has an unworn example of 'Lena Lastik hygienic underwear' with the price label still attached. These close-fitting combinations in cream coloured wool and elastic, have a straight neckline with rayon ribbon straps and are daintily edged with rayon lace and ribbon. In 1919 Dickins and Jones' fine merino combinations sold at 9/11, while another similar example, the Braemar, retailed for 19/6 c.1939. Killerton's collection also includes a pair of combinations in smart peach-coloured knitted rayon with a fancy knitted top. They are similar to those offered as 'lace designs' by Dickins and Jones in their pre-war 'Economy Week' catalogue of March 1939, when prices were cut from 21/9 to 13/9 for a pair of lightweight spun silk combinations.

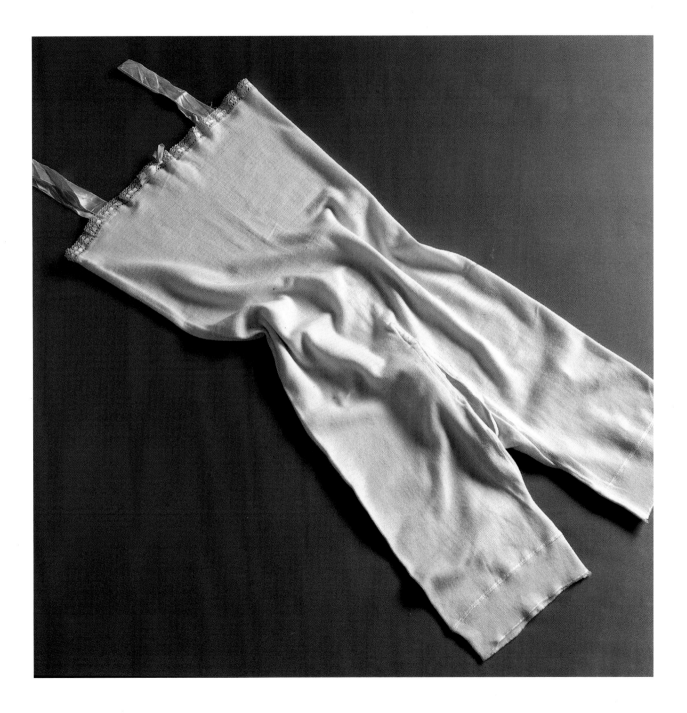

The 1930s - the Sylph and Synthetics

These delicate camiknickers – combined camisoles and knickers – of flimsy peach chiffon and black lace are examples of the sheer underwear that was worn under the fitted dresses of the 1930s and 40s.

❧

By the 1930s, only the older generation wore the traditional voluminous styles in white cotton. Close-fitting synthetic brassières and knickers, slips and knitted combinations were favoured by the fashionable and were essential to provide a smooth line underneath fitted and slinky dresses. Girdles could provide extra support – in fact many did not feel decently dressed without one, and they certainly would have given a smooth line under the bias-cut dresses which clung to the hips. Expensive, hand-finished lingerie in silk, lace and chiffon was also available throughout the 1920s and 30s and much of the underwear that survives from this period is amazingly flimsy and sheer.

Bras were particularly lightweight. 'The new brassières…are more necessary than ever with the new curved line and they are quite an item to buy. Why not make them yourself…' suggests *Economy in the Home*, published by the Singer Sewing Machine Company in the early 1930s. Another Singer booklet, *Save and Have* (c.1928), proposed recycling the tops of good silk stockings as 'a distinctive brassière' suitable for evening wear or warm weather. A more expensive but still minimal set of underwear was purchased for Flower Roberts, later Lady Furness, to wear under her wedding dress in 1930. Made of cream silk edged with Honiton lace, the simply cut bra top and knickers are finely embroidered with a horseshoe and blue ribbons.

A new rival was emerging for the corset companies: the fitness movement. Organisations such as the Women's League of Health and Beauty promoted the idea of shaping the body through a good diet and regular exercise, and magazines like *Good Housekeeping* published articles on overcoming obesity and emaciation. Advertisers claimed that 'a woman's most treasured possession today is the graceful slimness which fashion decrees', and more suspiciously, that 'figures in the public eye keep slim and trim on Vitawheat'. The sylph-like figure appeared increasingly in advertising – for instance, for the Kestos brassière.

With the rise of Hollywood and the increased influence of stage and screen, glamour became the essential tool in marketing lingerie. Articles such as 'On Screen and Stage' in a special lingerie issue of *Roma's Pictorial* in February 1934 reinforced the link. Free patterns were included for a complete set of lingerie – nightdress, petticoat, chemise, knickers and brassière – illustrated on the front cover. Synthetic materials were recommended, and the magazine advertisements could provide plenty of suggestions, such as the Courtaulds range, 'guaranteed to wash and wear'.

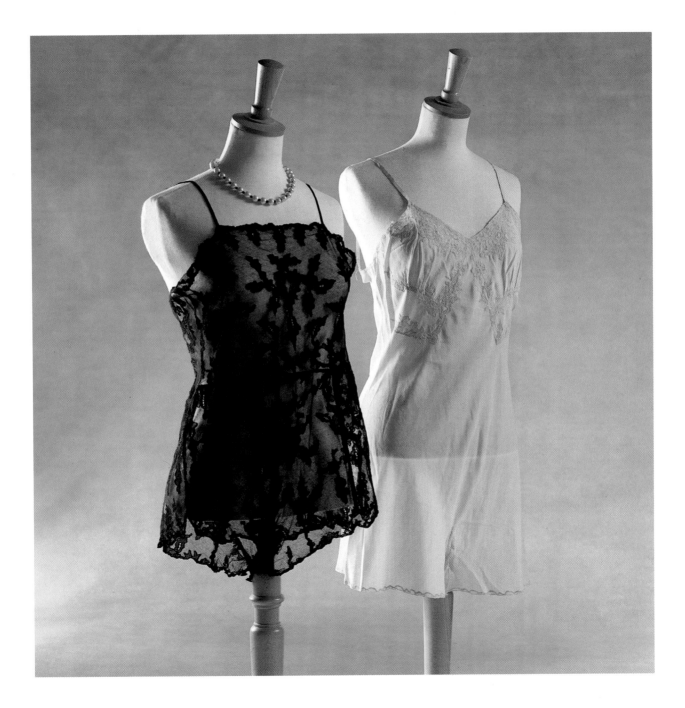

Wartime and New Look

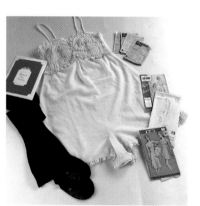

With the coming of the Second World War the emphasis was laid on prolonging the life of clothes rather than buying new and squandering scarce resources. Textiles and clothing disappeared as factories were turned over to the making of valuable supplies for the war effort, such as parachute manufacture. Clothes rationing was introduced in 1941 along with the utility mark. Clothing coupons were 'spent' carefully and darning was a virtue.

Government publications and advice in the media counselled careful washing and mending, as certain commodities were extremely scarce. Undergarments could be sewn from recycled clothes or hand-knitted at home. Some materials, such as lace, were off ration and could therefore be used for lingerie and trousseau nightwear without the need for coupons. Killerton has a few examples of underwear and nightwear made from parachute nylon. Patterns showed how to lay out the pieces and get the most from each panel.

New girdles were not available in the shops, therefore advertisements placed by firms such as Berlei were intended to remind magazine readers of the brand name until production was restored after the war. Stockings, particularly the new nylons, were famously available on the black market. Instead of bare legs, women wore short socks or tinted their skin with leg make-up known as 'liquid stockings'. There are some who claim to have used tea to stain their legs, carefully drawing a stocking seam down the back of the leg with an eyebrow pencil.

Rationing continued into the early 1950s, and even then some items were in short supply, as most manufacturers concentrated their efforts on supplying the export market. The 'New Look' launched by Christian Dior in 1947 caused great excitement, not least because it demanded a new type of girdle reminiscent of the lines of the Victorian and Edwardian corset. The 'Waspie' encouraged a tiny waist, and was set off by the extravagant full skirts of Dior's Corolle line. The look was to last well into the 1950s, and spawn anew developments in textile innovations and designs for underclothing. Recent developments in textile manufacture, such as nylon and versions of rayon, created a new market for easy care and washable garments which went hand in hand with the post-war boom and the demand for washing machines and specialist detergents.

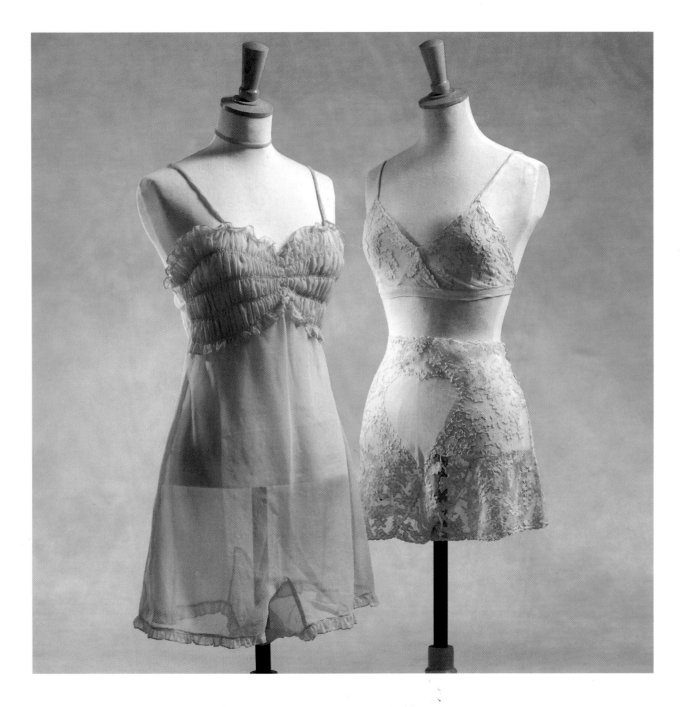

Select Bibliography

BOOKS

Adburgham, Alison, *Shops and Shopping 1800–1914*, Allen and Unwin, 1964

Ashelford, Jane, *The Art of Dress*, The National Trust, 1996; paperback edition 2000

Ashelford, Jane, *Care of Clothes*, The National Trust, 1997

Bradfield, Nancy, *Costume in Detail 1730–1968*, Harrap, 1968

Carter, Alison, *Underwear: The Fashion History*, Batsford, 1992

Cunnington, C.W. and P., *The History of Underclothes*, Michael Joseph, 1951, revised edition, Faber & Faber, 1991

Earnshaw, Pat, *Lace in Fashion*, Batsford, 1985

Ewing, Elizabeth, *Dress and Undress: A History of Women's Underwear*, Batsford, 1978, paperback edition 1989

Farrell, Jeremy, *Socks and Stockings*, Batsford, 1992

Foster, Vanda, and Walkley, Christina, *Crinolines and Crimping Irons; Victorian Clothes: How they were cleaned and cared for*, Peter Owen, 1978

Leroy, Ernest, *Le Corset à travers les Ages*, Paris, 1893

Levitt, Sarah, *Victorians Unbuttoned: Registered Designs for Clothing, their Makers and Wearers, 1839–1900*, Allen and Unwin, 1986

Newton, Stella Mary, *Health, Art and Reason: Dress Reformers of the Nineteenth Century*, John Murray, 1974

Ribeiro, Aileen, *Dress and Morality*, Batsford, 1986

Waugh, Norah, *Corsets and Crinolines*, Batsford, 1964; paperback edition 1987

ARTICLES

Alden, Maureen, 'The Beguilement of Zeus – In all the Better Shops' *Costume* No. 33, 1999

Arnold, Janet, 'Elizabethan and Jacobean Smocks and Shirts' *Waffen und Kostumkunde* vol.12, 1977

Mactaggert, P. and R.A., 'Half a Century of Corset Making: Mrs Turner's Recollections' *Costume* No.11, 1977

Mactaggert, P. and R.A., 'Ease, Convenience and Stays 1750–1850' *Costume* No.13, 1979

Sorge, Lynn, 'Eighteenth-Century Stays: Their Origins and Creators' *Costume* No.32, 1998

CONTEMPORARY JOURNALS AND MAGAZINES, SHOP CATALOGUES AND PATTERNS

La Belle Assemblée (1806–1840s)

The Workwoman's Guide (1838)

The Englishwoman's Domestic Magazine (1860s)

The Queen (1861 onwards)

The Girl's Own Paper (1880–1920s)

The Lady (1885 onwards)

Home Chat (1895 onwards)

Vogue (published in Britain from 1916 onwards)

Weldons Pattern Books (1890s–1930s)